The Low Carb Cookbook For Beginners

How to Lose Weight with Quick and Healthy Low Carb Diet Recipes
Bonus: 45 Days Weight Loss Challenge

1st Edition

Julia Sophie Harris

TABLE OF CONTENTS

i

TABLE OF CONTENTS

iii

TABLE OF CONTENTS

TABLE OF CONTENTS

v

The author's ideas and opinions contained in this publication serve to educate the reader in a helpful and informative manner. We accept the instructions may not suit every reader and we expect the recipes not to gel with everyone. The book is to be used responsibly and at your own risk. The provided information in no way guarantees correctness, completion, or quality. Always check with your medical practitioner should you be unsure whether to follow a low carb eating plan. Complete elimination of all misinformation or misprints is not possible. Human error is not a myth!

Our food is nutrients, and the three primary nutrients are carbohydrates, proteins, and fats. We may choose to favour or restrict any of these macronutrients, which allows us to classify diets as high-carb, low-fat, high-protein, or low-carb. When we restrict carbs to under 130g per day, we are talking about a diet that is low in carbohydrates. What happens when we are on a low-carb diet? And how low-carb can we go?

When we eat fewer carbs, we must supply the rest of the calories that the body needs to make fuel from the other two sources: fat and protein. Thus, a low-carb diet is a diet high in protein and healthy fats. Why do people choose to eat more fat and reduce carbs? Isn't that against common sense? Well, no. Fats have always been blamed for obesity, perhaps because being obese literally means being fat.

Based on that belief, low-fat foods were invented to minimize obesity and make all people slender. In reality, the so-called low-fat foods were the beginning of the obesity epidemics because, while they were deprived of all fats, those foods were packed with all the bad carbs. Since they are less calorie-rich, it is easy to eat more carbs than your body needs. So, what happened to the extra carbs? The body turned them into fat.

People go for low-carb diets because they want to shed weight. How does it work? Sugar and starches, i.e., carbohydrates, make our blood sugar levels oscillate and tend to heighten insulin (fat-storing hormone) levels. At some point, the body can no longer produce enough insulin to normalize blood sugar levels, i.e., we get Type 2 diabetes. Therefore, if we take starches and sugar away, we get stabilized blood sugar levels and reduced insulin levels.

We get a balance. We stay away from obesity, and we lose weight because the body must feed on something. We are not giving the body carbs, so it must feed on fat and protein. Plus, the body will not feel like it needs to eat as much since glucose levels are stabilized and they don't go up and down triggering hunger all the time.

Carbs are the most abundant form of biomolecules, and they are mainly responsible for transporting energy. Carbohydrates are informally referred to as carbs and are starches or sugars. Carbs are an essential food source. However, they become a problem when we give our body too many carbohydrates. In fact, we give our body so many that the it can't store them as glycogen and must turn them into fat. Too many carbs make us fat.

Did you know that...?

- Carbohydrates, carbs or saccharides are the same thing.

- Main sources of starch are bread, rice, pasta, beans, and cereals.

- Fruits are mostly sugars, and sugars are carbohydrates.

- High glycaemic index (GI) carbs enter the bloodstream as glucose.

- A low-GI diet improves the chance of a healthy lifestyle and weight.

TYPES OF CARBOHYDRATES

1. **Monosaccharides:**

   Monosaccharides are the smallest sugar units. Glucose is energy for the cells. Galactose is found in milk and dairy. Fructose is found in vegetables and fruit.

   - Glucose

   - Galactose

   - Fructose

2. Disaccharides:

Disaccharides are carbs that form by bonding two molecules of monosaccharides.

- Lactose (glucose + galactose)

- Maltose (glucose + glucose)

- Sucrose (glucose + fructose)

3. Polysaccharides:

Polysaccharides are a chain of two or more monosaccharides. Glycogen is a polysaccharide that humans and animals store in the liver and muscles.

Simple and complex carbs

1. Simple carbs

Monosaccharides and disaccharides are simple carbs. On the other hand, polysaccharides are complex carbs. Sugars are simple carbs, and they are a rapidly absorbed form of fuel or energy. However, while the effect of elevating blood sugar levels is quick, the drop of blood sugar levels and the increase in insulin levels is just as quick. Essentially, when we eat sugars, we feel satiated for a very short time. Hunger sets in quickly after.

2. Complex carbohydrates

Complex carbs are long-chain sugar molecules. Basically, wholegrains are the best examples. Since they have fibre still attached to sugars, complex carbs fill us up for longer. That's why fruit, wholemeal pasta, or vegetables are considered healthier than simple carbs, such as candies, even though they are still sugars.

NUTRITION

When we take on a low-carb diet, we are told by the sceptics that the brain cannot burn fat, and so it needs glucose that comes from burning carbs. But fewer carbs does not mean zero carbs and a low-carb diet is rich in good carbs, plenty for the neurons to burn.

The body turns carbohydrates immediately into glucose for energy. It also stores some carbs in the liver as glycogen for future use. The extra carbs intake that the body does not use immediately or store for later becomes fat. But what happens when we don't provide the body with enough carbs to make fuel for its processes? When not provided enough carbs, the body turns to other sources of energy, such as fat and protein. As a result, the body starts burning the fat we give it as well as the fat it has stored for fuel.

Scientifically, fewer carbs stabilize glucose levels and reduce the need for the pancreas to produce huge amounts of insulin to be able to bring down the high glucose levels that high carb intake produces. A drop of the insulin levels minimizes fat storage in the body, which stimulates weight loss. Long-term, the body will need more and more insulin to reduce glucose levels. It's called insulin resistance. At some point, the pancreas's beta cells will be depleted of insulin, and insulin will have to be provided from external sources. In short, you've got diabetes.

Cutting carbs is linked to what is often called low-carb flu. The symptoms may include dizziness, irritability, headaches, weakness, and nausea. These may be called withdrawal symptoms because they are a manifestation of the body's addiction to carbs as a source of energy. Our body has no experience in using anything but carbs as fuel, especially not fats. It has always burnt carbs for fuel.

However, these symptoms typically go away in days or weeks. Some of these symptoms become more evident for people who exercise regularly. Why? It's a new thing for the body to burn fat or protein for fuel. As such, it takes longer for the body to access fat as fuel, which makes fat a slower source of energy. In time, the body adapts, and the symptoms go away.

A low-carb diet is not a zero-carb diet. There are plenty of good carbs out there. When calculating carb intake, nutritionists don't look at total carbs as reference; they look at net carbs and dietary carbs. Net carbs end up as sugars in our body. In nature, foods are not high in net carbs, not even net carb packed veggies or fruits exceed 30% in net carbs. However, processed foods do exceed 30% in net carbs, and that's where the problem is. Those are the carbs that we need to cut down on a low-carb diet. The problem is not eating a fruit that is high in carbs but has mostly dietary carbs. The problem is eating processed foods that are high in net carbs that come from added sugars.

Eating low-carb is eating fewer carbs than fat or protein. But what does it literally mean as far as the foods we eat, our everyday meals? How restrictive is a low-carb diet? What is good for us and what should we keep our hands off? Here is what you CAN eat while on a low-carb diet:

MEATS

The first rule of low-carb diet is simple: stay away from processed foods. Meat is one of the most heavily processed foods in our diets. The second rule: check the source. When people eat meat, they often forget where it comes from, i.e., actual animals. The way the animals are raised is what gives meat its quality. Essentially, we can eat all meats on a low-carb diet if the meat is not processed and comes from reliable sources. However, it's best to maintain a balance between protein and fat intake.

SEAFOOD AND FISH

You can include seafood and fish in your low-carb diet, and you don't have to worry about your carb intake. Fish is preferred for so many reasons and the most popular of choices is fatty fish, including mackerel, salmon, and tuna.

EGGS

Eggs are considered a stable low-carb food. Versatile, nutritious, and packed with good fats, eggs can suit any preference. However, not all eggs are created equal, and, it is important that you consume eggs that come from grass-fed hens. People have different tolerance when it comes to eggs. As with all things in life, try and maintain a balance and stick to 3-6 eggs per day.

FRUIT

A low-carb diet is not compatible with a high fruit intake. Fruit are packed with a lot of carbohydrates and, in most fruits, that's sugar not dietary fibre. However, you can still include some low-carb fruits in your low-carb diet. are compatible with a low-carb diet if you keep your daily net carb intake under control. Fruit with low-carb content include raspberries, avocados, melons, and tomatoes.

Use an app to calculate your net carbs. Make a meal plan and see how many net carbs you are eating and how many of them come from fruit and veggies. When you realize how much sugar comes from fruits, you will know what to cut down.

NON-STARCHY VEGGIES

Unlike starchy veggies, such as potatoes, non-starchy veggies grow above the ground. Leafy greens occupy the first positions in the top of preferences for low-carb dieters. You can include successfully spinach, lettuce, green beans, broccoli, and other similar veggies in your low-carb diet. Not to mention that non-starchy veggies are incredibly versatile when it comes to cooking. You can consume many of them raw or cook them to replace high net carb foods such as pasta or rice.

HIGH-FAT DAIRY

With an abundance of low-fat or diet dairy products, people have started to forget how proper Greek yogurt even tastes. What people don't know is that the fat in those products must be replaced by something and that something is sugar; not just any sugar, but simple sugars that are rapidly absorbed and lead to diabetes. So, on a low-carb diet, feel free to consume full-fat dairy products such as brie, cheddar cheese, mozzarella, crème fraiche, soured cream, double cream, butter, and more. Stay away from margarine though. Mind the overall calorie intake but choose high-quality full-fat dairy products.

NUTS

Nuts are one of the best sources of plant-based fats. They are compatible with a low-carb diet. However, mind the quantity. It's very easy to consume nuts in excess since they are small and very tasty. Use in salads or occasional snacks. Plus, just like not all carbs are created equal, not all nuts are low-carb. Whole nuts, pecans, and macadamia are best, while cashew nuts are at the opposite end. As always, moderation is key.

DRINKS

A low-carb diet allows you to drink as much water as possible. Unsweetened coffee is also allowed and there are no restrictions except your personal preferences. If you choose a low-carb, high-fat diet, you can have a bullet proof coffee which is fortified with MCT oil, butter, or coconut oil.

Unsweetened tea is also a great choice and so is bone broth. The tea variety is entirely up to you. Drink as much as you like if you are not adding any sugars or artificial sweeteners. Hydrating, filling, and complete with nutrients and electrolytes, bone broth is a great way to increase your liquids intake while you are on a low-carb diet.

SUGARS

Sugars are carbs so essentially you need to stay away from them. You will discover that sugar is a hidden ingredient in so many products that it's unbelievable. Read labels if you do buy pre-packed foods. Stay away from all fruit juice (you only need a glass to exceed your net carb intake)! Mostly, forget about soft drinks, sports drinks, and other similar drinks. As for actual foods, forget about chocolate, candy, cakes, cookies, or any sweets all together, including maple syrup or agave syrup. From condiments to sauces and dressings, sugar is everywhere. Again, check the labels. You will soon discover the brands you can trust and those you can't.

STARCHES

Starches are the second biggest but equally important restriction in a low-carb diet. Main sources of starches are bread, pasta, rice, or muesli. Don't think that wholegrains are better. They are better than simple carbs, but they are still carbs so you must keep your hands off them as well! Also, legumes, such as lentils and beans, have a high carb content. On the other hand, some root vegetables, such as swede or celery root, are acceptable.

OTHER

Beer is packed with rapid-absorption carbs. It is essentially liquid bread so stay away from ear. Also, stay away from margarine, a heavily processed product. Switch to olive oil, butter, and other sources of healthy fats

First, should you pay attention to net carbs or total carbs? Net carbs are obtained by extracting dietary fibre from total carbs. Since dietary fibre is good for you, it is obvious why you should be concerned about your net carb intake, not your total carb intake. The only reason you need to look at total carb is to make sure you get enough dietary fibre. As mentioned earlier, high net carb foods are typically processed foods and starches, such as potatoes, rice, pasta, etc.

- A **keto diet:** is a low carb diet where net carb intake is under 20g of net carbs per day.

- A **moderate low-carb diet:** net carb intake is 20 to 50g per day.

- A **liberal low-carb diet:** net carb intake between 50 and 100g per day.

Strictly speaking, any diet with a carb intake lower than 130g per day is a low-carb diet. It's incredibly easy to achieve 130g of carbs a day. For example, 150 g of grapes contains 25g of net carbs. A cup of pasta contains 31g of net carbs. It's unbelievable how many carbs we put in our bodies and it is no wonder that the body cannot consume it all immediately or store it in the liver for future use. So, it turns it into fat. And, that is the most simplistic rationale behind a low carb diet.

KNOW YOUR FOOD

Starting a low-carb diet begins with understanding nutrients, i.e., our food. You must understand what you eat and how what you eat affects your body. You shouldn't look at carbs as the enemy but rather as something you can live without. There are essential amino acids (proteins) and essential fats (fatty acids) but there are no such things as essential carbs, are there?

KEEP TRACK OF NET CARBS

A good way to start with a low-carb diet is to use an app that helps you calculate you net carbs. There are many out there. You only need to find the one that suits you best. Next, you must understand what you cannot eat and how eating those foods impacts your net carb intake. After you plan a day carefully to stay under your target net carb intake and you have an apple at the end of the day, you will feel very disappointed to find out that you have completely failed to achieve your goal with just one apple So, include the apple in the diet in the first place, and still stay under your target.

SHOP LOW-CARB

Next, you must plan your meals a week ahead so you can shop accordingly. You must have everything you need in house, so you have no excuse for failing to complete the challenge. Most importantly, don't buy the no-noes of a low-carb diet: processed foods, sweets, juices, sodas, etc. If you keep a bowl of fruit on the table and you've been a vegan all your life, i.e., high-carb dieter, it's difficult to resist temptation since fruit is a staple food for vegans.

BE PREPARED FOR RESISTANCE

It is also important to be physically and emotionally prepared to give up carbs. You will experience withdrawal-like symptoms: fatigue, dizziness, nausea, headaches, sore muscles, etc. And, be prepared for your workouts to be crappy for a while. Fat and protein are not as easily accessible as fuel as crabs are. Plus, the body resists. It doesn't want to give up that easy way of making energy.

Time: 30 minutes | Serves: 4

Ingredients:

♦ 2 tbsps. olive oil
♦ 75 g minced beef
♦ 2 free-range eggs
♦ 60 g grated coloured cheddar cheese
♦ Small, square baking tray

Preparation:

1 Heat your oven to 200°C (400°F).

2 Heat oil in a pan over moderate heat. Add the minced beef to the pan. Fry until brown.

3 Place the cooked beef in the baking dish. Create two holes and crack in the eggs. Spread an even layer of cheddar cheese on top.

4 Place the tray with the beef, eggs, and cheese in the oven. Allow 15 minutes for the beef and beef to cook. Remove the tray from the oven and set aside for 10 minutes to cool.

Net carbs: 2 g | Fibre: 0 g | Fat: 36 g | Protein: 42 g | Kcal: 509

Time: 10 minutes | Serves: 1

Ingredients:

- 80 g avocado
- 1 hardboiled egg
- 1tbsp. olive oil
- 25 g brie cheese
- 20 g lettuce
- 100 g plum tomatoes
- 8 green olives (pitted)
- 50 g firm tofu
- Salt and pepper to taste

Optional:
- Pickled jalapenos
- Fresh parsley (chopped)

Preparation:

1. Heat ½ of the oil in a small sauce pan. Add the tofu and cookon both sides until golden brown. Remove from heat and transfer to cutting board. Let cool.

2. Meanwhile, cube the avocado, brie, and hard-boiled egg. Add to a medium-sized bowl. Finely chop the lettuce and cut the plum tomatoes in halves. Add them to the bowl.

2. Cube the tofu and add the cubes to the bowl along with the green olives and remaining olive oil. Mix to combine. Season with salt and pepper and decorate with parsley. Add in sliced jalapenos for a hot morning!

Net carbs: 4.53 g | Fibre: 3 g | Fat: 43 g | Protein: 20 g | Kcal: 504

Time: 5 minutes | Serves: 1

Ingredients:

♦ 180 ml coconut milk
♦ 25 g chia seeds
♦ ½ tsp vanilla extract

Preparation:

1 Place ingredients in an air-tight glass bowl. Mix well to combine. Secure lid and place in the fridge overnight for the seeds to gel.

2 Serve pudding for breakfast topped with coconut cream and fresh raspberries!

3 Serving suggestions! Stir in a touch of cinnamon, nut butter or cocoa butter for a different flavour!

Net carbs: 7 g | Fibre: 8 g | Fat: 44 g | Protein: 7 g | Kcal: 461

Time: 20 minutes | Serves: 2

Ingredients:

♦ 4 free-range eggs
♦ 225 g spinach leaves (chopped)
♦ 25g + 50 g butter
♦ 180 g diced streaky bacon lardons
♦ 30 g pecans
♦ 60 ml frozen cranberries
♦ Salt and pepper

Preparation:

1   Heat 50 g of the butter over moderate heat in a medium-sized frying pan. Add in the chopped spinach and fry until wilted. Remove spinach from pan.

2   Add the streaky bacon lardons to the same sauce pan. Fry the bacon pieces until they become crispy. Use a spatula to stir occasionally. Reduce heat. Add the wilted spinach, frozen cranberries, and pecans to the pan. Stir for the ingredients to combine and allow 1-2 minutes for ingredients to warm through. Remove from pan.

3   Increase heat to moderate and place remaining 25g of butter in the same pan. Crack the eggs into the pan. Cook to preference. Season with salt and pepper.

4   Transfer eggs to plates. Add a portion of the spinach, bacon, cranberries, and pecans mix. Enjoy immediately!

Net carbs: 8 g | Fibre: 6 g | Fat: 99 g | Protein: 26 g | Kcal: 1033

BACON AND SPINACH OMELETTE

Time: 15 minutes | Serves: 4

Ingredients:

- Low-carb sandwich:
- 4 tbsps. butter
- 4 eggs
- 225g cottage cheese
- 150 g smoked ham, slices
- 150 g cheddar cheese, slices
- 1 tbsp. ground psyllium husk powder
- *Salad:*
- 120 g lettuce
- ½ tbsp. lemon juice
- 4 tbsp olive oil
- salt and pepper

Preparation:

1. **Batter for "toast":** crack the eggs in a medium-sized bowl and whisk them until frothy and smooth. Incorporate the ground psyllium husk powder and cheese gently until you have a lump-free batter. Let rest for 5 minutes.

2. Heat 1 tbsp. of butter in a medium-sized saucepan over moderate heat. Add ¼ of the batter to the pan, like a pancake. Fry for 2 minutes. Flip and fry on the other side for 2 more minutes. Repeat for 3 more pancakes.

3. **Sandwich:** Using the pancakes as substitute for "toast", put together a sandwich with egg toast, ham, and cheese.

4. **Salad:** Mix the chopped lettuce with olive oil and lemon juice and season with salt and pepper! Divide the salad and arrange on plates. Enjoy warm!

Net carbs: 8 g | Fibre: 4 g | Fat: 92 g | Protein: 54 g | Kcal: 1082

Time: 50 minutes | Serves: 4

Ingredients:

♦ 900 g swede (peeled, cubed)
♦ 900 g chicken thighs (boneless)
♦ 1 tbsp. paprika
♦ salt and pepper, to taste
♦ 120 g butter

For serving:
♦ 240 ml creme fraiche

Preparation:

1 Heat your oven to 200°C (400°F). Split the chicken quarters and place them in a baking dish.

2 In an oven-proof tray, place the chicken thighs and cubed swede. Season to preference with the paprika powder and salt and pepper. Cube or slice the butter and place on top uniformly.

3 Place the tray in the oven and allow 40 minutes for the chicken and swede to cook through. Give it a shake halfway. Remove from heat.

4 Serve hot with crème fraiche!

Net carbs: 15 g | Fibre: 6 g | Fat: 103 g | Protein: 40 g Kcal: 1165

Time: 25 minutes | Serves: 4

Ingredients:

♦ 200 g unsmoked bacon rashers
♦ 120 g button mushrooms (finely sliced)
♦ 650 g minced beef
♦ Salt and pepper to taste
♦ 100 g grated cheddar cheese
♦ 1 iceberg lettuce

Preparation:

1 **Bacon:** Heat a saucepan over moderate heat. Add the bacon and fry to preference. Transfer bacon to a plate. Reserve the rendered fat.

2 **Mushrooms:** Fry the mushroom slices in the bacon fat for 5 minutes. Remove from pan and set aside.

3 **Beef:** Add salt and pepper to minced beef and mix to combine. Add the beef to the pan and allow 10 minutes to cook through. Use a spatula to break up chunks.

4 **Wraps:** Separate the lettuce leaves. Use a spoon to place equals amounts of the minced beef into lettuce leaves to make 4 servings. Top with the cheddar cheese, mushrooms, and crispy bacon. Serve with chopped fresh parsley!

Net carbs: 5 g | Fibre: 2 g | Fat: 51 g | Protein: 48 g | Kcal: 684

LOW CARB CHEESY MINCED BEEF WRAPS

Time: 50 minutes | Serves: 6

Ingredients:

- ♦ 120 g butter
- ♦ 1 yellow onion (peeled and finely chopped)
- ♦ 2 garlic cloves (minced)
- ♦ 450 g minced beef
- ♦ 1 red bell pepper (finely chopped)
- ♦ 225 g swede (peeled, cubed)
- ♦ 1 tbsp. dried oregano
- ♦ 1 tbsp. paprika powder

- ♦ 1 tsp. salt
- ♦ ¼ tsp. cayenne pepper
- ♦ ¼ tsp. ground black pepper
- ♦ 400 g cubed tomatoes (canned)
- ♦ 1½ tsp. red wine vinegar
- ♦ 700 ml water

Preparation:

1. Heat the butter in a medium-sized frying pan over moderate heat. Add in the minced garlic and finely diced onions and sauté until softened.

2. To the same pan, add the minced beef and let brown while breaking the chunks with a wooden spatula. Allow to cook through.

3. Add seasonings, swede cubes, and bell pepper and let simmer for 1 more minute stirring to combine. Add the diced tomatoes and 2/3 of the water.

4. Turn up heat and bring to a gentle boil. Allow 10 more minutes for the soup to simmer. Stir in the vinegar and remaining water until well combined. Remove from heat.

5. Serve hot with soured cream. Decorate with fresh parsley. Enjoy!

Net carbs: 11 g | Fibre: 4 g | Fat: 42 g | Protein: 16 g | Kcal: 491

Time: 25 minutes | Serves: 4

Ingredients:

- 2 tbsp butter
- 150 g diced bacon
- 2 garlic cloves (minced)
- 1 yellow onion (julienned)
- 225 g celery root (peeled and diced)
- 225 ml water
- 450 ml double cream
- 1 cube fish-flavoured bouillon
- 1 tbsp. white wine vinegar
- 1 tbsp. fresh thyme (finely chopped)
- 1 bay leaf
- 225 g ready-to-eat mussels
- salt and pepper

Preparation:

1   Heat butter in a medium-sized frying pan over moderate heat. Add in bacon and fry until very crispy. Transfer the bacon to a plate. Reserve the bacon grease.

2   In the same pan, sauté the garlic, onions, and celery root until golden. Stir in the thyme and bay leaf.

3   Add the heavy cream, fish-flavoured bouillon cube, water, and vinegar to the pan. Bring to a light boil. Reduce hit and allow 10 minutes to simmer.

4   Finely, add the mussels. Stir and allow the chowder to simmer for 2 more minutes. Check for saltiness before seasoning. Mussels can be salty. Remove from heat and set aside.

5   Serve hot in soup bowls topped with fried bacon and chopped parsley.

Net carbs: 12 g | Fibre: 2 g | Fat: 65 g | Protein: 19 g | Kcal: 708

Time: 20 minutes | Serves: 2

Ingredients:

- 50 g cottage cheese
- 1 tbsp. fresh chives
- 60 ml mayonnaise
- 1 green bell pepper (finely sliced)
- 2 avocados (pitted, wedged)
- 1 yellow onion (finely sliced)
- 75 g kale (finely chopped)
- 4 free-range eggs
- 3 tbsp.extra virgin olive oil
- salt and pepper

Preparation:

1   Place the mayo and cottage cheesein a mixing bowl. Add in the chives and season with salt and pepper. Mix until well combined.

2   Place the olive oil in a medium-sized frying pan over moderate heat. Add the julienned onions, chopped kale, and sliced bell peppers. Let cook until golden brown. Season with salt and pepper.

3   Make four holes in the greens and crack the eggs. Season with salt and pepper. Lower heat and let the eggs cook to preference. Remove from heat.

4   Serve the greens and egg with cottage cheese. Enjoy!

Net carbs: 14 g | Fibre: 17 g | Fat: 81 g | Protein: 21 g | Kcal: 897

Time: 40 minutes | Serves: 2

Ingredients:

♦ 250 g cauliflower florets
♦ 150g broccoli florets
♦ 70 g softcheese
♦ 75 ml double cream
♦ 75 grated cheddar
♦ 20 g butter
♦ salt and pepper
♦ 1 tsp. garlic powder
♦ 5" baking dish

Preparation:

1   Heat your oven to180°C (350°F).

2   Add the broccoli florets to a pot boiling salty water and let cook until fork tender. Strain and place in a mixing bowl. Discard water.

3   Add the double cream, soft cheese and seasonings to boiled broccoli florets. Use a hand mixer to mash to a smooth consistency.

4   Use the butter to grease generously the baking tray. Place the cauliflower florets on the bottom. Cover with the cream and broccoli sauce. Top with grated cheddar.

5   Place the oven-proof tray in the oven and allow 40 minutes to bake. The cheese should have turned a dark golden colour.

Net carbs: 6 g | Fibre: 2 g | Fat: 56 g | Protein: 36 g | Kcal: 675

Time: 55 minutes | Serves: 4

Ingredients:

- ♦ 2 garlic cloves (peeled)
- ♦ 2 shallots (peeled, cut into wedges)
- ♦ 300 g rutabaga (peeled and cubed)
- ♦ 300 g pumpkin (peeled and cubed)
- ♦ 2 tbsps. olive oil
- ♦ 225 g butter

- ♦ ½ litre vegetable broth
- ♦ Juice of ½ lime
- ♦ Salt and pepper to taste

For serving:
- ♦ 180 ml crème fraiche
- ♦ 35 g pumpkin seeds (roasted)

Preparation:

1   Heat your oven to 200°C (400°F).

2   Add the cubed pumpkin, cubed rutabaga, shallot wedges and garlic cloves to an oven-proof dish. Drizzle with the olive oil. Season to taste. Place the tray in the oven. Let the veggies roast for 30 minutes until fork tender. Remove from oven.

2   Transfer the roasted vegetables to a pot. Pour the vegetable stock on top. Place the pot on moderate heat and bring to a gentle boil. Lower heat and simmer for 5 minutes more. Remove from stove.

3   Add the cubed butter, seasonings, and lime juice to the soup. Use a hand blender to puree the soup to a smooth consistency.

4   Serve in soup bowls with crème fraiche and roasted pumpkin seeds!

Net carbs: 14 g | Fibre: 3 g | Fat: 88 g | Protein: 6 g | Kcal: 865

Time: 35 minutes | Serves: 4

Ingredients:

♦ 50 g butter
♦ 225 ml double cream
♦ 600 g green beans
♦ 75g grated cheddar cheese
♦ 300 g smoked rashers bacon
♦ salt and pepper

Preparation:

1 Heat oven to 200°C (400°F).

2 Heat butter in a frying pan over moderate heat. Add the green beans to the pan and let cook until tender. Transfer green beans to baking tray and season with salt and pepper. Set aside.

3 Place the double cream in a saucepan over moderate heat. Bring to a light boil. Reduce heat and stir in the grated cheddar to incorporate. Continue to stir until the cheddar has completely melted. Season with salt if needed. Stir in pepper to taste.

4 Transfer the mixture to the baking tray in a uniform layer. Let cook for 20 minutes. the colour should be a dark gold. Remove from oven and set aside to cool for 5 minutes.

5 While the creamy green beans are cooking, place the bacon in a frying pan over moderate heat. Fry to desired crispiness.

6 **Serving:** Transfer the creamy green beans to plates. Top with crispy bacon and finely chopped fresh chives.

Net carbs: 7 g | Fibre: 3 g | Fat: 91 g | Protein: 45 g | Kcal: 1030

Time: 10h15 minutes | Serves: 4

Ingredients:

♦ 600 g beef for roasting
♦ 2 tbsp. Avocado oil
♦ 60 g radishes (quartered)
♦ 60 g carrots (sliced)
♦ ¼ large yellow onion (julienned)
♦ 1 sprig fresh thyme
♦ 1 sprig fresh rosemary
♦ 160 ml beef broth

Preparation:

1 Season the meat to taste by rubbing in the salt and pepper all sides. Set aside to rest at room temperature for 40 minutes.

2 Place ½ of the avocado oil in a thick-based pot over moderate-high heat. Add in the onion and cook until golden. Next, add the quartered radishes and sliced carrots and let brown, not soften, for 5 more minutes. Remove from pot and set aside.

3 Transfer the seasoned beef to the pot with 1 tablespoon of oil. Brown the meat on all sides. Remove from pot and transfer to slow cooker. Arrange the veggies evenly around the meat. Pour the beef broth and add the thyme and rosemary springs halfway into the broth.

4 Set the timer to 5-6 hours on high or 10-12 hours on low. The meat should be very tender when done. Serve with soured cream sprinkled with finely sliced chives!

Net carbs: 2 g | Fibre: 2 g | Fat: 19 g | Protein: 29 g | Kcal: 307

CROCK-POT LOW CARB BEEF AND VEGGIES

Time: 3h15 minutes | Serves: 4

Ingredients:

- 4 medium-sized chicken breasts
- 4 garlic cloves (minced)
- 1 tbsp. olive oil
- 225 ml double cream
- 80 ml chicken broth
- 180 g parmesan cheese (grated)

- Salt and pepper
- 1 tbsp. Italian seasoning
- 180 gr baby spinach (chopped)
- ½ cup sun-dried tomatoes (chopped)

Preparation:

1 Place a medium-sized frying pan over medium heat. Add the oil and garlic gloves. Use a spatula to spread the garlic evenly in the pan and let sauté until fragrant.

2 Pour the chicken stock and double cream over the garlic and bring it to a simmer. Reduce heat to low and let it cook for 10 minutes. Add the Parmesan progressively while stirring until melted and combined. Season to taste. Remove from heat.

3 Season chicken breasts by rubbing in the Italian seasonings on all sides. Place the breasts in the centre of the slow cooker and sprinkle with the chopped sun-dried tomatoes.

4 Pour the cheese sauce over the chicken breasts. Set the timer on 6-8 hours on low or 3-4 hours on high. Remove chicken breasts from the cooker and transfer to plates.

5 Increase heat to high on the slow cooker. Add in the spinach and let it cook for a couple of minutes until wilted while stirring. Turn off and set aside.

4 Top the chicken breasts with the cheese and spinach sauce and decorate with freshly chopped parsley.

Net carbs: 8 g | Fibre: 1 g | Fat: 35 g | Protein: 45 g | Kcal: 542

RECIPES FOR DESSERTS

Time: 15+15 minutes | Serves: 4

Ingredients:

♦ 60 g coconut flour
♦ 6 free-range eggs (large)
♦ 180 ml coconut milk (unsweetened, canned)
♦ 2 tbsp. coconut oil (melted)
♦ 5 g (1 tsp.) baking powder
♦ Salt to taste
♦ Butter for frying
♦ Fresh berries for serving

Preparation:

1   Place egg yolks and egg whites in two separate bowls. Use a hand mixer to beat the egg whites with a bit of salt to a firm consistency. Set aside.

2   Add the coconut oil and coconut milk to the egg yolks and beat until well combined. Gently incorporate the flour and baking powder until it forms a smooth batter. Fold in the whisked egg whites. Set aside to rest for 5 minutes.

3   Heat the butter in a frying pan over moderate heat. Scoop in the batter and fry the pancakes for 1-2 minutes on each side.

4   Serving suggestion! Serve pancakes with crème fraiche and fresh berries.

Net carbs: 3 g | Fibre: 8 g | Fat: 24 g | Protein: 12 g | Kcal: 291

Time: 35 minutes | Serves: 12

Ingredients:

♦ 240 ml double cream
♦ 1/2 tsp. vanilla extract
♦ 45 g unsalted butter (room temperature)
♦ 45 g dark chocolate (chopped)
♦ 9 x 9 cm tray

Preparation:

1 Preparation tip! Place the double cream in a thick-based saucepan over moderate-high heat. Stir the vanilla extract into the double cream and bring to a gentle boil. Lower the heat. Let simmer while stirring occasionally until the double cream has reduced to half the initial amount.

2 Incorporate the room temperature butter until you achieve a smooth batter. Remove pan from heat and set aside. Stir the chocolate into the hot mixture until completely melted and well combined.

3 Pour the batter into your ray. Place in the fridge for 2 hours.

4 Remove tray from the fridge. Use a fine strainer to sprinkle a uniform layer of cocoa powder on top. Cut the chocolate fudge into 12 pieces and serve one piece as dessert!

Net carbs: 2 g | Fibre: 2 g | Fat: 12 g | Protein: 1 g | Kcal: 118

Time: 40 minutes | Serves: 6

Ingredients:

- ◆ Cinnamon-spiced apples
- ◆ 1 tsp. ground cinnamon
- ◆ 3 medium apples (tart and firm)
- ◆ 3 tbsp.unsalted butter

Vanilla sauce
- ◆ ½ tsp vanilla extract
- ◆ 600 ml double cream
- ◆ 1 egg yolk
- ◆ 2 tbsp. unsalted butter

Preparation:

1   **Cinnamon apples:** Remove the core of each apple and slice them finely. Heat butter in a frying pan over moderate heat. Add the apples and cook until golden-brown. Towards the end, sprinkle in the cinnamon and stir to coat the apples evenly. Remove from heat and set aside.

3   **Vanilla sauce:** Make the vanilla sauce a day ahead! Place the butter, vanilla extract, and ¼ of the double cream in a saucepan over moderate heat. Bring to a gentle. Reduce heat and let simmer. Continue to stir for 5 more minutes until a creamy consistency is achieved. Remove from heat.

4   Incorporate the egg yolk while mixing the sauce vigorously. Place in the refrigerator and let cool completely.

5   In a separate bowl, add remaining double cream and whisk to a firm consistency. Soft peaks should form. Fold gently into the refrigerated vanilla sauce. Place in fridge and let cool for 30 more minutes.

6   **Serving:** Place the vanilla cream sauce into serving bowls or cocktail glasses. Top with the cinnamon apples!

Net carbs: 12 g | Fibre: 2 g | Fat: 47 g | Protein: 4 g | Kcal: 476

Time: 5 minutes | Serves: 4

Ingredients:

- ♦ 2 tsp. olive oil
- ♦ 225 g full-fat soft cheese
- ♦ fresh parsley, chopped
- ♦ Zest of ½ lemon
- ♦ 1 garlic clove, minced
- ♦ 4 celery stalks, rinsed and cut to desired length
- ♦ salt and pepper

Preparation:

1   **Preparation tip!** Substitute parsley with fresh or dried herbs of choice, including fresh basil, fresh dill, or dried oregano.

2   Place the thick soft cheese in a medium-sized bowl. Incorporate remaining ingredients except the celery stalks until well combined. Season to taste and mix some more. Place the soft cheese mixture in the fridge for at least 10 minutes.

2   **Serving suggestion!** Serve the herbed soft cheese with celery stalks or other low-carb vegetable sticks, such as cucumber or bell pepper sticks.

Net carbs: 5 g | Fibre: 1 g | Fat: 22 g | Protein: 4 g | Kcal: 229

Time: 15 minutes | Serves: 4

Ingredients:

- ♦ 12 mini bell peppers (red, orange, and yellow)
- ♦ 240 g soft cheese (full-fat)
- ♦ 30g chorizo sausage (finely diced or thinly sliced)
- ♦ 1 tbsp. fresh coriander (finely chopped)
- ♦ ½ tbsp. chipotle paste (mild or hot)
- ♦ 2 tbsp. olive oil

Preparation:

1 **Preparation tip!** Substitute the coriander with any fresh or dried herbs of choice: parsley, thyme, dill, or basil!

1 Cut the mini peppers lengthwise in halves. Remove the seeds and the core and arrange on a serving platter.

2 Place the soft cheese into a small mixing bowl. Add the olive oil, chorizo, and herbs and mix until well combined. Season with chipotle paste!

3 **Serving suggestion!** Place an equal amount of the soft cheese mixture into each of the 12 mini bell peppers.

Net carbs: 7 g | Fibre: 1 g | Fat: 29 g | Protein: 6 g | Kcal: 311

Time: 5 minutes | Serves: 2

Ingredients:

220 g berries of choice, fresh

1 tbsp. lime juice

400 ml coconut milk (unsweetened, canned)

½ tsp. vanilla extract

Preparation:

1   Place the solid part of the canned coconut milk in a blender.

2   Add the berries, vanilla extract, and lime juice to the blender.

3   Pulse to desired smoothness.

4   **Serving suggestion!** Serve with fresh mint and a sprinkle of chia seeds!

Net carbs: 10 g | Fibre: 1 g | Fat: 42 g | Protein: 5 g | Kcal: 418

Time: 10 minutes | Serves: 6

Ingredients:

15 g cocoa powder

750 ml coconut milk (canned, unsweetened)

1 tsp vanilla extract

Preparation:

1   **Preparation tip!** Place the coconut milk cans in the fridge and let sit overnight. Refrigeration separates the milk into coconut water and solid cream.

2   Use a fine drainer to separate the solid coconut cream from the water. Set the coconut cream aside in a mixing bowl.

3   Add vanilla extract and cocoa powder to the coconut cream bowl. Use a hand-held mixer to whisk the ingredients until well combined.

4   **Serving suggestion!** Place an equal amount of the mixture into 6 serving bowls. Decorate with fresh mint leaves or 3-5 fresh raspberries.

Net carbs: 4 g | Fibre: 1 g | Fat: 28 g | Protein: 3 g | Kcal: 260

REFRESHING LOW-CARB CHOCOLATE MOUSSE

The only way to be successful on a diet is to not be on a diet. Confusing? Most likely. The point is that we can only succeed to reap the benefits of a certain diet if we stop seeing it as a diet. If we see the benefits of a diet is healthy additions to our lifestyle, we stop associating the diet with restrictions. A low-carb diet, whether you go for keto, moderate, or liberal, is not as restrictive as other diets. It's certainly a doable diet and can be adopted as a long-term lifestyle with great advantages to our health.

If you arm yourself with a 45-day low-carb meal plan, you are most likely to succeed. Our 45-day low-carb challenge is easy to follow since it's focused on foods you can easily buy. Plus, you don't have to be a chef to prepare any of the recipes. They are very easy to make. Hopefully, at the end of this challenge, you will get a better understanding of food and how it affects you. You may discover that cooking can be fun and easy, and you may choose to do it everyday for the benefits it offers to you and your family.

Starting a low-carb challenge is about being prepared with the ingredients you will need to make your meals. Also, it's about getting rid of all the bad carbs in your cupboard. In addition, you must be prepared for potential low-carb flu symptoms and some not-so-good workouts in the first week or two. Otherwise, a challenge is exactly that: a challenge. It implies a certain level of effort and ambition.

Enjoy your food!

Breakfast

Blueberry coconut milk smoothie

Time: 5 minutes | Serves: 2
Net carbs: 10 g | Fibre: 1 g | Fat: 43 g | Protein: 4 g | Kcal: 415

Ingredients:

♦ 125 ml frozen blueberries
♦ 1 400 g-can coconut milk
♦ 1 tbsp. lemon juice
♦ ½ tsp. vanilla extract

Preparation:

1   Use a blender to mix all ingredients to a creamy, smooth consistency.
2   Add more lemon juice if necessary!

Lunch

One-pot roasted chicken thighs and swede

Dinner

Comforting Pumpkin Soup

DAY 1

Breakfast

Hearty avocado salad

Lunch

Quick spinach and salmon plate

Time: 5 minutes | Serves: 2
Net carbs: 1 g | Fibre: 0.7 g | Fat: 89 g | Protein: 32 g | Kcal: 1022

Ingredients:

♦ 325 g smoked salmon
♦ 225 ml mayonnaise, divided
♦ 60 g baby spinach
♦ 1 tbsp olive oil
♦ ½ lime (optional)
♦ salt and pepper

Preparation:

1 Divide salmon, baby spinach on plates. Place a wedge of lemon next to it. Spoon mayo on plates. Season the spinach and drizzle with olive oil!

2 Enjoy!

Dinner

Cauliflower and cheese casserole

Breakfast

Beef, eggs, and cheese morning casserole

Lunch

Low-carb cheesy minced beef wraps

Dinner

Rotisserie chicken and buttery green beans

Time: 15 minutes | Serves: 2
Net carbs: 5 g | Fibre: 3 g | Fat: 89 g | Protein: 48 g |Kcal: 1009

Ingredients:

♦ 450 g roast whole cooked chicken
♦ 200 g fresh green beans
♦ 75 g butter for serving
♦ salt and pepper

Preparation:

1   Heat the butter in a medium size pan over moderate heat. Add the green beans and let cook to desired doneness. Towards the end, season with salt and pepper.

2   Place the buttery green beans and chicken on a plate. Top with butter and serve immediately!

Breakfast

Breakfast tuna and avocado plate

Time: 15 minutes | Serves: 2

Net carbs: 3 g | Fibre: 7 g | Fat: 76 g | Protein: 52 g | Kcal: 931

Ingredients:

- ◆ 4 eggs, boiled to taste
- ◆ 50 g baby spinach
- ◆ 275 g tuna in olive oil
- ◆ 1 avocado (pitted, sliced or diced)
- ◆ 125 ml mayonnaise
- ◆ ¼ lemon
- ◆ salt and pepper

Preparation:

1   Arrange the avocado, eggs, and tuna on plates. Top the tuna with ½ of the mayonnaise and lemon wedge.

2   Season with salt and pepper. Enjoy!

Lunch

Low-carb beef goulash

Dinner

Creamy green beans and crispy bacon

Breakfast

Chia seeds pudding

Lunch

Oven-roasted low-carb veggies and sausages

Time: 50 minutes | Serves: 4

Net carbs: 4 g | Fibre: 1 g | Fat: 43 g | Protein: 25 g | Kcal: 510

Ingredients:

- ♦ 450 g sausages
- ♦ 30 g butter, for greasing
- ♦ 2 yellow onions (wedged)
- ♦ 1 small zucchini (cubed)
- ♦ 3 garlic cloves (sliced)
- ♦ 150g cherry tomatoes
- ♦ 200 g mozzarella cheese (cubed)
- ♦ 60 ml olive oil
- ♦ Salt and pepper
- ♦ 1 tbsp. dried basil
- ♦ Soured cream for serving

Preparation:

1 Heat your oven to 200°C (400°F).

2 Coat an oven tray with butter. Set aside.

3 Place the wedged onions, cubed zucchini, sliced garlic, whole cherry tomatoes, and mozzarella cubes in the oven tray. Sprinkle the dried basil over the veggies and mozzarella and season with salt and pepper.

4 Drizzle everything with olive oil. Place sausages on top. Transfer the tray to oven and let cook for 40 minutes. The sausages should be cooked through and the veggies caramelized. Remove from oven!

7 Serve immediately with soured cream.

Dinner

Crock-pot low-carb beef and veggies

DAY 5

Breakfast

Bacon and spinach omelette

Lunch

Low-carb mussels' soup

Dinner

Fried aubergines and anchovies' salad

Time: 30 minutes | Serves: 4
Net carbs: 9 g | Fibre: 8 g | Fat: 47 g | Protein: 15 g | Kcal: 532

Ingredients:

♦ 900 g aubergines, sliced lengthwise

♦ 3 tbsp. olive oil, for brushing

♦ 150 g mozzarella cheese (cubed)

♦ 200 g plum tomatoes (halved)

♦ 50 g anchovies in olive oil

♦ salt and pepper

Dressing:

♦ ½ lemon, juiced

♦ 125 ml olive oil, for dressing

♦ 1 garlic clove (minced)

♦ Finely chopped fresh parsley

Preparation:

1 Brush the eggplant slices with2 tbsps. of olive oil on each side and season to taste.

2 Heat a medium-sized frying pan over moderate heat. Add the eggplant slices and fry for 5 minutes on each side

while turning occasionally. Remove from heat.

3 In a small bowl, mix olive oil with the garlic, lemon juice, and parsley until well combined.

4 On a serving platter to fit all eggplant slices, pour the garlicky dressing. Arrange the aubergine slices on the dressing and allow 1 minute to absorb the dressing. Flip the aubergine slices.

5 Add the tomato halves, anchovies, and cubed mozzarella over the aubergine slices. Drizzle with lemon juice and the remaining olive oil from the anchovies and season to taste!

Breakfast

Cauliflower pancakes

Time: 30 minutes | Serves: 4
Net carbs: 5 g | Fibre: 3 g | Fat: 26 g | Protein: 7 g | Kcal: 278

Ingredients:

- ♦ 110g butter, for frying
- ♦ 450 g cauliflower (grated)
- ♦ 3 free-range eggs
- ♦ ½ yellow onion (minced)
- ♦ Salt and pepper

Preparation:

1. Place the grated cauliflower with remaining ingredients in a mixing bowl to fit all ingredients. Mix until well combined. Let sit for 10 minutes.

2. Heat a generous amount of butter in a pan over moderate heat. Add a scoop of the cauliflower batter (enough to form a 3-4 inches pancake) to the pan and flatten to form a 4-inch pancake. Reduce heat. Cook for 5 minutes on each side just like pancakes. Repeat to finish all batter.

3. Serve with crème fraiche!

Lunch

Low-carb creamy Tuscan chicken

Dinner

Cauliflower and cheese casserole

DAY 7

59

Breakfast

Low-carb pancakes

Lunch

Oven-roasted cauliflower and broccoli gratin

Time: 35 minutes | Serves: 6
Net carbs: 12 g | Fibre: 4 g | Fat: 42 g | Protein: 18 g | Kcal: 496

Ingredients:

- 1 leek (roughly chopped)
- 1 yellow onion (roughly chopped)
- 450 g broccoli florets (chopped)
- 225 g cauliflower florets (chopped)
- 450 g pre-cooked sausages (sliced)
- 50 g butter, for frying
- 2 tbsp. Dijon mustard
- 150 g grated cheese
- 240 ml crème fraiche
- Fresh thyme
- salt and pepper

Preparation:

1. Heat your oven to 225°C (450°F).

2. In a large frying pan, heat ½ of the butter over moderate heat and fry the onion, leeks, broccoli, and cauliflower. Remove from heat.

3. In a separate frying pan, heat remaining butter and fry the sausages. Remove from heat and set aside.

4. In a mixing bowl, mix the crème fraiche and Dijon mustard until well combined. Pout the mustard and crème fraiche mixture over the veggies.

5. Arrange the fried sausage slices over the mustard and cream sauce. Top with a uniform layer of grated cheddar. Season with salt and pepper and thyme.

6. Place the baking tray in the oven on the upper rack. Let bake for 15 minutes. Remove from oven! Enjoy!

Dinner

Comforting Pumpkin Soup

Breakfast

Soft cheese-stuffed mini bell peppers

Lunch

Greens and eggs skillet

Dinner

Low-carb broccoli soup

Time: 20 minutes | Serves: 4
Net carbs: 10 g | Fibre: 2.8 g | Fat: 54 g | Protein: 7.2 g | Kcal: 551

Ingredients:

- 1 leek (finely sliced)
- 300 g broccoli (florets)
- 1 vegetable bouillon cube
- ½ litre water
- 200 ml double cream
- 200 g cream cheese
- fresh basil
- 1 garlic clove (minced)
- Salt and pepper

Preparation:

1. In a medium-sized pot, add the broccoli florets and leeks. Cover with water and add the vegetable bouillon cube and a pinch of salt. Place the pot over high heat and allow to come to a boil. Let boil for 2 minutes so that broccoli is tender and bright green. Remove from heat!

2. Add in the double cream, soft cheese, garlic, basil, and black pepper. Use a hand blender to whisk to desired smoothness. Add water if too thick. Add double cream if too thin.

3. Transfer the soup to plates and serve with freshly chopped basil!

DAY 9

Breakfast

Ginger and spinach coconut cream smoothie

Time: 5 minutes | Serves: 2
Net carbs: 3 g | Fibre: 1 g | Fat: 8 g | Protein: 1 g | Kcal: 82

Ingredients:

- 2 tsp. fresh ginger (grated)
- 150 ml water
- 75 ml coconut cream
- 2 tbsp. lemon juice
- 30 g frozen spinach

Preparation:

1 Place all smoothie ingredients in a blender. Pulse to desired consistency. Add more or less lemon juice to accommodate your taste.

2 Serve with grated ginger1 Enjoy!

Lunch

One-pot roasted chicken thighs and swede

Dinner

Creamy green beans and crispy bacon

Breakfast

Low-carb ham and cheese sandwich

Lunch

Creamy courgette salad

Time: 15 minutes | Serves: 1
Net carbs: 8 g | Fibre: 7 g | Fat: 54 g | Protein: 8 g | Kcal: 556

Ingredients:

♦2 courgettes
♦1 tbsp. olive oil
♦salt and pepper
♦1Romaine lettuce head
♦110g rocket leaves
♦finely chopped fresh chives
♦¾ cup pecans (chopped)

Dressing
♦2 tbsp olive oil
♦175 ml mayonnaise
♦2 tsp. lemon juice
♦1 garlic clove
♦½ tsp. salt
♦¼tsp chili powder

Preparation:

1   Cut the courgette lengthwise. Remove seeds and slice crosswise in ½-inch pieces. Cut the romaine lettuce into bite-size pieces.

2   Add the zucchini pieces in a pan where the olive oil is shimmering over moderate heat. Season to taste and allow the zucchini pieces to fry until golden. Remove from heat.

3   In a salad bowl, place the rocket leaves, chopped lettuce, and chives. Place the romaine, arugula and chives in a large bowl. Add the sautéed courgette pieces and stir to combine.

4   Toast the pecans in the same pan as the courgette. Season to taste. Transfer into the salad bowl.

5   Mix dressing ingredients until well combined. Pour the mayo dressing over the courgette salad and toss to coat all ingredients with the creamy dressing. Enjoy!

Dinner

Low-carb cheesy minced beef wraps

Breakfast

Refreshing low-carb chocolate mousse

Lunch

Low-carb beef goulash

Dinner

Creamy cabbage dinner casserole

Time: 60 minutes | Serves: 6
Net carbs: 11 g | Fibre: 4 g | Fat: 49 g | Protein: 11 g | Kcal: 527

Ingredients:

- 90 g butter, for frying
- 850 g green cabbage (shredded)
- 1 yellow onion (minced)
- 2 garlic cloves (minced)
- 300 ml double cream
- 80 ml soured cream
- 150 g full-fat soft cheese
- 150 g cheddar cheese (grated)
- Salt and pepper

Preparation:

1 Heat your oven to 200°C (400°F).

2 Place butter in a large oven-proof pan and heat over moderate-high heat. Add the onion, garlic, and cabbage. Stir to combine and allow 10 minutes to sauté.

3 When the cabbage has started to soften, add the double cream, soured cream, and soft cheese. Season to taste. Mix until well combined. Allow 5-8 minutes to simmer. Remove from heat.

4 Spread the mixture uniformly in the pan. Add the grated cheddar in an even layer over the cheese and veggie mixture. Place the pan in the oven. Bake for 15-20 minutes.

5 Transfer to plates and enjoy!

Breakfast

Bacon egg nests

Time: 20 minutes | Serves: 3
Net carbs: 1 g | Fibre: 0 g | Fat: 11 g | Protein: 16 g | Kcal: 171

Ingredients:

♦ 5 back bacon rashers
♦ 75 g crumbled mature cheddar
♦ 6 large eggs
♦ salt and pepper
♦ 6-cup non-stick muffin tray

Preparation:

1   Heat your oven at 200°C (400°F). Grease the wells of the muffin tray with butter or coat them with cooking spray.

2   Coat the muffin wells with the bacon rashers to form a bacon bowl. Add crumbled cheddar in each muffin well.

3   Crack the eggs into the wells. Season to taste. Place in the oven for 12 to 15 minutes for the eggs to set.

4   Remove from oven. Transfer to plates and serve immediately! Decorate with fresh parsley or fresh basil!

Lunch

Low-carb mussels' soup

Dinner

Crock-pot low-carb beef and veggies

Breakfast

Beef, eggs, and cheese morning casserole

Lunch

Coconut milk curried chicken thighs

Time: 30 minutes | Serves: 4

Net carbs: 10.25 g | Fibre: 3 g | Fat: 59 g | Protein: 25 g | Kcal: 612

Ingredients:

- 3 tbsp butter
- 1 yellow onion (julienned)
- 1 red chili pepper (finely sliced)
- 1 tbsp. fresh ginger (grated)
- 1 tbsp. red curry paste
- 450 g chicken thighs (boneless,

skinless)
- 100g green beans (fresh, sliced to desired length)
- 225 g broccoli florets (small)
- 750 g coconutmilk
- salt and pepper, to taste

Preparation:

1. Heat butter in a wok over moderate heat. Add the onion, chilli pepper, and ginger to the pan. Allow 5 minutes to fry until fragrant.

2. Slice the chicken thighs into thin strips. Add to the wok along with the curry paste. Stir until well combined. Allow 5-8 minutes for the chicken to brown. To avoid burning the chicken, stir in more butter.

3. Add the small broccoli florets and sliced green beans to the work. Separate the solid coconut cream from the coconut water and add the solid cream to the work. Season to taste. Lower heat and allow 15-20 minutes to simmer.

4. Transfer to plates and serve hot! Enjoy!

Tip! Keep the coconut milk cans in the fridge for 4 hours prior to using. It helps separate the solids from liquid.

Dinner

Low-carb creamy Tuscan chicken

Breakfast

Hearty avocado salad

Lunch

Low-carb mussels' soup

Dinner

Stir-fried cauliflower rice Indonesian style

Time: 20 minutes | Serves: 2
Net carbs: 15 g | Fibre: 6 g | Fat: 62 g | Protein: 18.5 g | Kcal: 698

Ingredients:

- 110 gbutter or olive oil
- 450 g cauliflower rice
- ½ green bell pepper (finely sliced)
- ½ yellow onion (finely sliced)
- 50 g green onions (finely sliced)
- 1 red chili pepper (finely sliced)
- 2 garlic cloves (minced)
- 30 g fresh ginger (grated)
- 4 free range eggs
- 1 tbsp.sesame oil
- salt and pepper

Preparation:

1   Heat the butter in a large pan over moderate to high heat. Add the scallions, onion, bell pepper, chilli, and cauliflower rice to the pan. Stir to combine. Fry until slightly golden.

2   Add the grated ginger and minced garlic to the pan. Stir to combine. Reduce heat and pour in the sesame oil. Season to taste. Stir to combine.

3   Crack the four eggs over the cauliflower mixture. Allow 1 minute to set. Stir to combine. Allow eggs to cook through.

4   Remove from heat and serve hot!

Breakfast

Spinach on egg toast

Time: 15 minutes | Serves: 1

Net carbs: 8.8 g | Fibre: 6.1 | Fat: 41 g | Protein: 21 g | Kcal: 500

Ingredients:

- 2 tbsps. olive oil
- ½ small red onion (finely chopped
- 1 garlic glove (minced)
- 180 g baby spinach (chopped)
- ¼ can low-sodium chopped
- tomatoes
- 2 free range eggs
- Finely chopped fresh dill
- 3 walnut halves
- Salt and pepper

Preparation:

1. Heat ½ of the olive oil over medium heat in a medium-sized work. Add the chopped red onion and minced garlic. Stir. Fry until the garlic is fragrant and onion is translucent.

2. Add the chopped spinach and stir to combine. Cook until the spinach has slightly wilted. Add the chopped tomatoes to the pan and stir. Season to taste. Increase heat and let simmer for 5 more minutes. Remove from heat and transfer to a strainer placed over a bowl for the excess liquid to drain.

3. Add remaining olive oil to a non-stick work over moderate high heat. whisk the eggs until frothy and smooth. Season to taste. Stir in the finely chopped dill and whisk until well combined. Pour the eggs into the wok and let the eggs coat the bottom in an even layer. Let fry until the eggs are nearly set. Flip. Cook for half a minute more. Remove from heat.

4. Place the spinach mixture in the middle of the omelette. Top with crushed walnuts and enjoy immediately!

Lunch

Greens and eggs skillet

Dinner

Cauliflower and cheese casserole

Breakfast

Chia seeds pudding

Lunch

Low-carb Swedish casserole

Time: 40 minutes | Serves: 6
Net carbs: 8.3 g | Fibre: 0.75 g | Fat: 62 g | Protein: 42 g | Kcal: 760

Ingredients:

- 2 tbsp. butter
- 225 g streaky bacon lardons (diced)
- 250 g chestnut mushrooms (sliced)
- 1 banana (peeled and sliced)

- 1 whole roasted chicken (deboned and shredded)
- 475 ml double cream
- 1 tsp. curry powder
- 125 ml mild chili sauce
- salt and pepper

- Preparation:

1 Heat your oven to 200°C (Mark 6 for gas oven or 400°F).

2 Heat butter in a medium-sized frying pan over moderate heat. Add the mushrooms slices to the pan. Stir in the =bacon. Fry to desired doneness. Season to taste. Remove from heat and transfer to a greased oven-proof tray.

3 Top the mushrooms and bacon with an even layer of the shredded chicken. Place banana slices over the chicken.

4 Using a hand mixer, mix the double cream until firm. Fold in the curry powder and chilli sauce, and season to taste. Place an even layer of the double cream mixture over the mixture in the tray.

5 Place in oven and allow 25 minutes to bake. Remove from oven and serve immediately!

Dinner

Comforting Pumpkin Soup

Breakfast

Bacon and spinach omelette

Lunch

One-pot roasted chicken thighs and swede

Dinner

Creamy beef stroganoff on courgette fettucine

Time: 30 minutes | Serves: 4
Net carbs: 12 g | Fibre: 3 g | Fat: 64 g | Protein: 40 g | Kcal: 788

Ingredients:

- 3 tbsp. butter
- 1 yellow onion (medium, finely chopped)
- 225g mushrooms (sliced to preference)
- 1 tbsp. dried thyme
- 350 ml full-fat soured cream
- 225 g Stilton blue cheese

- (crumbled)
- 450 g minced beef
- Salt and pepper
- Courgette pasta:
- 2 courgettes (julienned lengthwise)
- 30 g olive oil
- salt and pepper

Preparation:

1 Sauté the onion until translucent in the butter in a medium pan over moderate heat. Add the minced beef to the pan and fry. Use a spatula to break the chunks. Let the meat fry until browned and cooked through.

2 Add the sliced mushrooms to the pan. Stir to combine with the onion and meat and allow 2 minutes to sauté. Add the crumbled blue cheese and soured cream and stir to combine. Bring to a gentle boil. Reduce heat and allow the mixture to simmer for 10 minutes. Remove from heat.

3 While the meat cooks, add the courgette slices to a pot of boiling salted water. Let the courgette boil for 1 minute. Drain the courgette slices, arrange on plates, and drizzle abundantly with the olive oil. Season to taste!

4 Serve the creamy beef mixture next to or on top of the zucchini slices! Enjoy!

DAY 18

Breakfast

Rich low-carb beef and cheese breakfast plate

Time: 5 minutes | Serves: 2

Net carbs: 5.35 g | Fibre: 5.5 g | Fat: 56.5 g | Protein: 38.5 g | Kcal: 695

Ingredients:

- 200 g deli roast beef
- 150 g mild cheddar cheese (sticks)
- 1 avocado (pitted, halved, and sliced)
- 6 radishes (trimmed, halved)
- 1 green onion spring (finely chopped)
- 4 tbsps. crème fraiche
- 1 tbsp Dijon mustard
- 2 tbsp. olive oil
- 50g lettuce (coarsely chopped)
- salt and pepper

Preparation:

1   Arrange the roast beef slices, avocado slices, cheddar sticks, and radishes on plates. Add the mustard and crème fraiche, and sprinkle with sliced green onions.

2   Mix lettuce and drizzle with olive oil! Divide and place on plates. Enjoy!

Lunch

Low-carb cheesy minced beef wraps

Dinner

Creamy green beans and crispy bacon

Breakfast

Low-carb ham and cheese sandwich

Lunch

Low carb baked brie

Time: 15 minutes | Serves: 4

Net carbs: 1.55 g | Fibre: 1.05 g | Fat: 30.05 g | Protein: 15 g | Kcal: 337

Ingredients:

♦ 250 g Brie round
♦ 1garlic clove (minced)
♦ 60g walnuts (chopped)
♦ 1 tbsp. olive oil
♦ 1 tbsp. fresh parsley (finely chopped)
♦ salt and pepper

Preparation:

1 Heat your oven to 200°C (mark 6 on gas or 400°F). Line a sheet pan with baking paper and set aside.

2 In a small bowl, mix the chopped walnuts, chopped parsley, minced garlic, and olive oil. Season with salt and pepper.

3 Arrange the cheese on the sheet pan. Transfer the nut and garlic mixture over of the brie cheese. Place the sheet pan in the oven. Bake for 10 minutes. Serve warm! Enjoy!

Dinner

Crock-pot low-carb beef and veggies

Breakfast

Vanilla cream and cinnamon apples bowls

Lunch

Low-carb beef goulash

Dinner

Low-carb halloumi dinner plate

Time: 15 minutes | Serves: 4
Net carbs: 4.3 g | Fibre: 5 g | Fat: 47 g | Protein: 18 g | Kcal: 518

Ingredients:

- ◆ 2 tbsp. butter
- ◆ 275 g halloumi cheese (4 slices)
- ◆ 2 avocados (pitted, sliced)
- ◆ ¼ cucumber (cut into sticks)
- ◆ 2 tbsp. olive oil
- ◆ 75 ml soured cream
- ◆ 2 tbsp. pistachio nuts
- ◆ salt and pepper

Preparation:

1   Melt butter in a medium frying pan over moderate heat. Fry the halloumi cheese slices on both sides until golden brown, about 2 minutes on each side. Remove from heat and transfer to plates.

2   Arrange the avocados, pistachios, and cucumber sticks on plates next to the cheese. Spoon in the soured cream. Drizzle the veggies with olive oil. Season with salt (if necessary) and freshly ground black pepper.

Breakfast

Low-carb bacon breakfast plate

Time: 15 minutes | Serves: 4
Net carbs: 4 g | Fibre: 8 g | Fat: 50 g | Protein: 14.5 g | Kcal: 534

Ingredients:

♦ 150 g streaky bacon rashers
♦ 4 eggs
♦ 2 tbsp butter, for frying
♦ 2 avocados (pitted, quartered)
♦ 1 green bell pepper (finely sliced)
♦ 30 g rocket leaves
♦ 4 tbsp. walnuts
♦ 2 tbsp. olive oil
♦ Salt and pepper

Preparation:

1   Melt butter in a saucepan over moderate heat. Add the streaky bacon rashers and fry to desired crispiness. Remove from pan. Reserve grease.

2   Reduce heat. Crack the eggs in the same pan in the fat rendered by the bacon. Fry to preference. Remove from pan and transfer to plates. Reserve fat.

3   Add the avocado quarters, bell pepper sticks, walnuts, and rocket leaves to plate. Sprinkle veggies with olive oil. Season to taste. Drizzle the eggs with the bacon fat.

Lunch

Low-carb mussels' soup

Dinner

Low-carb creamy Tuscan chicken

Breakfast

Bacon and spinach omelette

Lunch

Low-carb asparagus and fried salmon

Time: 15 minutes | Serves: 2
Net carbs: 2 g | Fibre: 2 g | Fat: 52 g | Protein: 28 g | Kcal: 591

Ingredients:

♦ 250 g salmon (2 fillets)
♦ 75 g butter
♦ 225 g green asparagus (trimmed)
♦ salt and pepper

Preparation:

1 Melt ½ of the butter in a large saucepan over moderate heat. Add the trimmed asparagus. Fry the asparagus for 4 minutes until tender but not soft. Season with salt and pepper. Move to one side of the pan.

2 Add ½ of the remaining butter and fry the salmon fillets in the empty side of the frying pan. About 2 minutes on each side should do it. Stir the asparagus occasionally as the salmon is frying.

3 Transfer to plates and season to taste if necessary. Top the fried salmon fillets with the rest of the butter.

Dinner

Greens and eggs skillet

Breakfast

Moderate low-carb berries smoothie

Lunch

Cauliflower and cheese casserole

Dinner

Swiss sauce ribeye steak

Time: 25 minutes | Serves: 6
Net carbs: 2 g | Fibre: 0.6 g | Fat: 66 g | Protein: 29 g | Kcal: 730

Ingredients:

Salad
- ◆50 g rocket leaves
- ◆50 g lettuce (coarsely chopped)
- ◆225 g baby plum tomatoes, halved

Swiss sauce
- ◆4 egg yolks
- ◆300 g butter (melted, lukewarm)
- ◆2 tsp. white wine vinegar

- ◆2tbsps. fresh tarragon (finely chopped)
- ◆½ tsp. onion powder
- ◆salt and pepper

Steak:
- ◆2 tbsps. butter
- ◆6 small ribeye steaks
- ◆salt and pepper

Preparation:

1   **Sauce:** Whisk the egg yolks with a hand mixer until creamy and smooth. Incorporate the lukewarm melted butter progressively as you increase speed. Add in the onion powder, tarragon, and vinegar. Season to taste.

2   Heat butter in a medium frying pan over moderate heat. Add ribeye steaks to pan. Fry the steaks on both sides to preference. Season to taste. Remove from heat and transfer to plates.

3   Mix the ingredients for the salad and transfer to plates next to the steaks. Pour a generous amount of the sauce over the steaks. Enjoy!

Breakfast

Low-carb cheesy mushroom omelette

Time: 10 minutes | Serves: 1

Net carbs: 4 g | Fibre: 1 g | Fat: 43 g | Protein: 25 g | Kcal: 510

Ingredients:

- ◆ 30 g butter
- ◆ 3 eggs
- ◆ 25 g Gouda cheese (1 slice)
- ◆ 3 mushrooms (finely sliced)
- ◆ ¼ small yellow onion (julienned)
- ◆ salt and pepper

Preparation:

1   In a small bowl, whisk eggs with a fork until frothy and smooth. Season to taste. Whisk the eggs into a mixing bowl. Season to taste.

2   Heat a medium-sized frying pan and melt butter. Pour the eggs and spread uniformly in the pan. Let eggs cook until almost eggs. They should still be raw on top.

3   Place the gouda slice in the middle and top with the mushroom slices and julienned onion. Fold the omelette over in half. Allow 20 seconds more to cook. Flip over and allow 20 seconds more to brown. Slide the omelette on a plate!

Lunch

One-pot roasted chicken thighs and swede

Dinner

Cauliflower and cheese casserole

DAY 25

Breakfast

Beef, eggs, and cheese morning casserole

Lunch

Oven-roasted creamy salmon fillets

Time: 15 minutes | Serves: 1

Net carbs: 8 g | Fibre: 5 g | Fat: 69 g | Protein: 41 g | Kcal: 822

Ingredients:

- 2 tbsps. olive oil
- 450 g broccoli florets
- 2tbsps. small capers
- 6 green onion springs
- 4 salmon fillets (700 g)

- 300 ml double cream
- Salt and pepper
- 1 tbsp. Dijon mustard
- 1 tbsp. dried parsley
- 90 g butter, slices

Preparation:

1   Heat your oven to 200°C (Mark 6 on gas or 400°F).

2   Heat olive oil on moderate heat in an oven-proof frying pan large enough to accommodate the veggies and fish. Add broccoli florets and cook for 5 minutes. Season to taste. Add the capers and green onion. Allow 2 more minutes to fry.

3   Remove from heat and arrange the salmon fillets among the veggies. In a separate bowl, mix double cream, parsley, and mustard, and add uniformly over the fish and veggies. Place the butter slices on top.

4   Transfer to oven and allow 20 minutes to cook. Remove from oven and transfer to plates!

Dinner

Low-carb ham and cheese sandwich

Breakfast

Comforting Pumpkin Soup

Lunch

Hearty avocado salad

Dinner

Low-carb tuna salad with poached eggs

Time: 20 minutes | Serves: 2

Net carbs: 6 g | Fibre: 3 g | Fat: 69 g " Protein: 29 g | Kcal: 765

Ingredients:

Tuna salad

- ♦ 110g tuna in olive oil (drained)
- ♦ ½ red onion (finely chopped)
- ♦ 1 tsp. Dijon mustard
- ♦ 125 ml mayonnaise
- ♦ Juice and zest of ½ lemon
- ♦ 2 tbsp small capers
- ♦ salt and pepper

- ♦ Poached eggs
- ♦ 1 tsp salt
- ♦ 2 tsps. white wine vinegar
- ♦ 4 free-range eggs

For serving:

- ♦ 75 g mixed lettuce leaves
- ♦ 75 g cherry tomatoes
- ♦ 2 tbsp olive oil

Preparation:

1   In a salad bowl, place all tuna salad ingredients. Combine well. Season to taste and transfer to fridge.

2   Stir in salt and vinegar in a pot of gently boiling water. Crack the eggs into the waters and allow 3 minutes for the whites to set. Transfer the eggs to a platter using a slotted spoon.

3   Spoon the tuna salad onto the plates. Mix salad ingredients and place on plates. Top the salad with the poached eggs. Seasonto taste!

DAY 27

Breakfast

Creamy salmon lettuce boats

Time: 20 minutes | Serves: 6
Net carbs: 3 g | Fibre: 0 g | Fat: 26 g | Protein: 23 g | Kcal: 330

Ingredients:

- 225 g full-fat soft cheese
- 200 g smoked salmon
- 80 ml mayonnaise
- Zest of ½ lemon
- Pepper to taste
- Finely chopped fresh dill
- 50 g lettuce in small boat-like leaves

Preparation:

1 Slice the smoked salmon into small pieces. Placein a bowlwith remaining ingredients except for the lettuce. Mix to combine. Allow 10-20 minutes for the flavours to set in.

2 Place the salmon salad on each lettuce leaf. Enjoy immediately!

Lunch

Chia seeds pudding

Dinner

Creamy green beans and crispy bacon

Breakfast

Bacon and spinach omelette

Lunch

Mussels and avocado lunch platter

Time: 15 minutes | Serves: 4

Net carbs: 3.5 g | Fibre: 7 g | Fat: 48 g | Protein: 17 g | Kcal: 525

Ingredients:

♦ 220 g ready-to-eat mussels (drained)
♦ 2 avocados (pitted, halved)
♦ 4 eggs boiled to preference
♦ 100 g cottage cheese
♦ 120 ml mayonnaise
♦ 40 g baby spinach leaves
♦ 2 tbsp olive oil
♦ salt and pepper

Preparation:

1   Arrange the avocados and eggs on serving plates. Add the mussels in small ramekins to the plate. Spoon the mayo and cottage cheese onto the plates.

2   Finely, slice the spinach leaves and drizzle with olive oil. Season to taste. Enjoy!

Dinner

Crock-pot low-carb beef and veggies

Breakfast

Low-carb ham and cheese sandwich

Lunch

Low-carb cheesy minced beef wraps

Dinner

Cold cuts dinner salad

Time: 10 minutes | Serves: 4
Net carbs: 12 g | Fibre: 9 g | Fat: 65 g | Protein: 38 g | Kcal: 821

Ingredients:

- ◆500 g iceberg lettuce (chopped)
- ◆freshly chopped parsley
- ◆150 g Italian ham
- ◆300 g mozzarella cheese (cubed)
- ◆150 g Italian salami
- ◆150 g roasted red peppers (canned, finely sliced)
- ◆300 g artichokes (canned, sliced)
- ◆120 g sun-dried tomatoes (finely sliced)
- ◆6 tbsp green olives

Dressing:
- ◆2 red chili pepper, finely chopped
- ◆8 tbsp olive oil
- ◆Finelychopped fresh basil
- ◆1 tbsp sea salt

Preparation:

1   Mix lettuce and parsley and arrange like a bed on a serving platter. Place the Parma ham and salami on top along with the cubed mozzarella. Spread remaining ingredients on top.

2   Mix dressing ingredients in a bowl. Drizzle over the salad! Serve immediately! Enjoy!

Breakfast

Low-carb fried eggs and bacon

Time: 10 minutes | Serves: 4

Net carbs: 1 g | Fibre: 0 g | Fat: 22 g | Protein: 15 g | Kcal: 272

Ingredients:

150 g smoked bacon rashers

8 free-range eggs

Baby plum tomatoes

Chopped fresh parsley

Preparation:

1 Add bacon to a pan and cook until crispy. Remove from pan. Reserve fat.

2 Add the eggs to the pan and fry to preference. While eggs cook, add the tomatoes to the pan and fry. Season to taste! Serve with chopped parsley!

Lunch

Low-carb beef goulash

Dinner

Low-carb creamy Tuscan chicken

Breakfast

Greens and eggs skillet

Lunch

Fried chorizo and roasted aubergines with avocado sauce

Time: 30 minutes | Serves: 4

Net carbs: 12 g | Fibre: 11 g | Fat: 82 g | Protein: 32 g | Kcal: 946

Ingredients:

Avocado sauce
- ♦ 1 avocado (pitted)
- ♦ 2 tbsps. water
- ♦ fresh parsley
- ♦ 3 tbsp. lime juice
- ♦ 1 green chili pepper
- ♦ 1 garlic clove (minced)
- ♦ 30 g pistachio nuts

- ♦ 75 ml. olive oil
- ♦ Salt and pepper

Chorizo and aubergines
- ♦ 900 g aubergines (4 aubergines)
- ♦ salt and pepper
- ♦ 3 tbsp olive oil
- ♦ 450 g chorizo sausage

Preparation:

1 Heat your oven to 200°C (400°F).

2 *Avocado sauce:* Place avocado sauce ingredients in a blender. Blend to desired consistency.

3 *Aubergines:* Cut the aubergines lengthwise. Use a brush to rub them with olive oil. Season to taste. Transfer to a baking sheet lined oven tray. Bake 20 minutes to roast. Aubergines must be soft.

4 *Sausage:* Heat a pan over moderate heat and fry the chorizo sausage to desired doneness.

5 Serve the chorizo sausage, halved aubergines, and avocado sauce! Decorate with fresh parsley!

Dinner

Low-carb mussels' soup

Breakfast

Low-carb pancakes

Lunch

Cauliflower and cheese casserole

Dinner

Creamy oven-baked bacon and brussels sprouts

Time: 15 minutes | Serves: 1
Net carbs: 4 g | Fibre: 1 g | Fat: 43 g | Protein: 25 g | Kcal: 510

Ingredients:

- ♦ 650g Brussels sprouts
- ♦ 5 garlic cloves (minced)
- ♦ 275 g bacon lardons (diced)
- ♦ 300 ml double cream
- ♦ 150 g grated cheddar cheese
- ♦ 60 g shaved parmesan cheese
- ♦ salt and pepper

Preparation:

1 Heat your oven to200°C (400°F).

2 Heat a medium-sized oven-proof pan over medium heat. Fry the bacon lardons to desired crispiness. Transfer the bacon to plates. Reserve grease.

3 Add the trimmed and quartered Brussels sprouts to the bacon grease. Add the garlic, stir, and fry the sprouts to desired tenderness.

4 Pour the double cream over the Brussels sprouts. Bring to a light boil. Reduce heat and allow 2 more minutes to simmer. Add the bacon and stir to combine.

5 Add the grated cheddar and parmesan in even layers over the cream, sprouts, and bacon mixture. Place in the oven and let bake for 10 more minutes.

Breakfast

Fried eggs with salsa and avocado

Time: 30 minutes | Serves: 1

Net carbs: 16 g | Fibre: 10 g | Fat: 51 g | Protein: 16 g | Kcal: 610

Ingredients:

♦ 2 tbsps. olive oil
♦ ½ yellow onion (finely chopped)
♦ ½ orange bell pepper (finely chopped)
♦ 2 garlic cloves (minced)
♦ 1 fresh jalapeño (minced)
♦ 1 tomato (peeled and diced)
♦ 2 free-range eggs
♦ ½ avocado (sliced)
♦ fresh parsley (finely chopped)

Preparation:

1. Heat 1 tbsp. of olive oil in a non-stick saucepan over moderate heat. Add the garlic, finely chopped onion, bell pepper, and minced jalapeño. Fry for 3 minutes while stirring. Add the diced tomatoes. Stir to combine and let cook for 5 more minutes.

2. In a separate non-stick saucepan, heat the remaining olive oil. Add the eggs and cook to desired doneness. Transfer eggs to plate.

3. Spoon the salsa onto the plate and add the avocado slices next to it. Decorate with freshly chopped parsley.

Lunch

One-pot roasted chicken thighs and swede

Dinner

Low-carb creamy Tuscan chicken

Breakfast

Vanilla cream and cinnamon apples bowls

Lunch

Dill and pepper sauce lamb stew

Time: 2h 10min | Serves: 6

Net carbs: 6 g | Fibre: 3 g | Fat: 49 g | Protein: 29 g | Kcal: 590

Ingredients:

- ◆ 900 g lamb shoulder (cubed)
- ◆ 2 bay leaves
- ◆ 1 tsp. white peppercorns
- ◆ 1 yellow onion (wedged)
- ◆ 1 carrot (sliced)

- ◆ Salt to taste
- ◆ 300 ml double cream
- ◆ 1 tsp. lemon juice
- ◆ fresh dill (finely chopped)
- ◆ 550 g fresh green beans

Preparation:

1. Place the cubed lamb shoulder into a pot of salted boiling water. Allow 5 minutes to boil on high heat. Remove from water and rinse. Set aside. Discard water.

2. Place the lamb cubes in the same pot. Add bay leaves, peppercorns, onion wedges, and sliced carrots. Add water to cover. Stir in salt and allow 2 hours to simmer.

3. Remove the cubed lamb from the broth and set aside. Use a strainer to strain the lamb stock. Discard boiled veggies. Return broth to pot and let boil until reduced to half.

4. Add the double cream to the broth. Bring the creamy broth to a boil. Let simmer for 15 minutes while stirring. Season to taste. Add in the lemon juice.

5. Return the meat to the pot. Simmer for a couple of minutes until the meat is warmed thorough. Season with the chopped dill.

6. Place the fresh beans in a pot of salted boiling water. Allow 4-5 minutes to boil. Remove from water and place onto plates. Serve with the dill and pepper sauce lamb stew.

Dinner

Comforting pumpkin soup

Breakfast

Beef, eggs, and cheese morning casserole

Lunch

Creamy green beans and crispy bacon

Dinner

Sugar snaps and egg sauce white fish

Time: 35 minutes | Serves: 4
Net carbs: 12 g | Fibre: 3 g | Fat: 68 g | Protein: 48 g | Kcal: 856

Ingredients:

Fish:
- 800 g white fish (cut into bite-size pieces)
- water

Egg sauce:
- 50 g butter
- 200 g cream cheese
- 325 ml double cream

- salt and pepper
- fresh parsley (chopped)
- 3 hardboiled eggs (chopped)

Serving:
- 2 tbsps. butter
- 450 g sugar snaps
- 1 lemon, sliced

Preparation:

1   **Fish:** Place the fish pieces in a saucepan. Cover with water. Place over high heat and let simmer for 3 minutes. Remove fish from water and keep warm. Discard water.

2   **Egg sauce:** Heat the butter in the same saucepan over moderate heat. When completely melted, add the double cream and soft cheese and stir to combine. Season to taste. Let simmer for 2 minutes while stirring continuously. Add the eggs and parsley and stir to combine. Remove from heat.

3   **Sugar snaps:** Heat the butter over moderate heat in a saucepan. Add the sugar snaps. Fry to desired tenderness.

4   Place the sugar snaps on plates. Add the fish pieces and smother with the eggs sauce.

Breakfast

South American chicken salad

Time:20 minutes | Serves: 4
Net carbs: 1 g | Fibre: 3 g | Fat: 30 g | Protein: 25 g | Kcal: 384

Ingredients:

- ♦ 450 g chicken breasts
- ♦ 2 tbsps. olive oil (divided)
- ♦ Salt to taste
- ♦ 225 ml water
- ♦

Sauce:
- ♦ 2 tbsps. mayonnaise
- ♦ 1 ripe avocado (pitted, chopped)
- ♦ fresh parsley (minced)

Preparation:

1 Heat ½ the olive oil in a medium size frying pan over moderate heat. Season chicken with salt and pepper and place into the pan. Allow 4 minutes to sear on each side.

2 Pour the water to the frying pan. Cover the pan and allow 5 minutes to simmer until the water has evaporated. Remove chicken from pan and set aside on a cutting board. Use two forks to shred it.

3 Toss all ingredients for the salad in a large bowl. Season to taste. Add the shredded chicken and mix lightly. Serve with freshly chopped parsley.

Lunch

One-pot roasted chicken thighs and swede

Dinner

Cauliflower and cheese casserole

Breakfast

Bacon and spinach omelette

Lunch

Oven-roasted garlic chicken

Time: 50 minutes | Serves: 4
Net carbs: 4 g | Fibre: 1 g | Fat: 39 g | Protein: 42 g | Kcal: 546

Ingredients:

♦ 4 tbsps. butter
♦ 900 g chicken drumsticks
♦ 5 garlic cloves (finely sliced)
♦ fresh parsley (finely chopped)
♦ Juice of 1 lemon
♦ 2 tbsp olive oil

Preparation:

1   Heat your oven to 225°C (450°F). use the butter to grease an oven-proof pan large enough to fit all drumsticks comfortably. Arrange the drumsticks in the pan. Sprinkle with parsley and garlic, and season to taste. Drizzle with the lemon juice and olive oil.

2   Transfer pan to the oven and allow 40 minutes to bake. Reduce temperature in the last 5 minutes. Remove from oven and transfer to plates. Serve with a leafy greens' salad or a cauliflower mash!

Dinner

Low-carb mussels' soup

Breakfast

Moderate low-carb berries smoothie

Lunch

Greens and eggs skillet

Dinner

Low-carb beef tenderloin with gravy

Time: 30 minutes | Serves: 4
Net carbs: 2 g | Fibre: 0 g | Fat: 60 g | Protein: 50 g | Kcal: 773

Ingredients:

♦ 150 g streaky bacon lardons (diced)
♦ ½ leek (finely sliced)
♦ 3 tbsps. butter
♦ 650 g beef tenderloin (4 steaks)
♦ 75 ml red wine
♦ 75 ml water
♦ salt or ground black pepper

Preparation:

1   Heat butter in a large pan over moderate heat. Add bacon lardons and leeks and fry to preference. Remove bacon and leeks from pan. Reserve the fat.

2   Add steaks to pan and fry 3 minutes on each side or to desired doneness. Remove from pan. Keep warm.

3   Add water and wine to the meat juices in the pan. Bring to a gentle boil. Allow to simmer to desired consistence. Strain for a lump-free gravy.

4   Place steak, bacon, and leeks on plates. Drizzle with gravy and enjoy! Serve with soured cream.

Breakfast

Deli turkey salad with creamy green sauce

Time: 10 minutes | Serves: 4
Net carbs: 12 g | Fibre: 3 g | Fat: 36 g | Protein: 26 g | Kcal: 482

Ingredients:

Salad
- 275 g baby plum tomatoes
- 275 g Romaine lettuce
- 75 g radishes
- 125 g green olives (pitted)
- 1 red onion
- 450 g deli turkey

Dressing
- 75 ml ready-made green salsa sauce
- 125 ml sour cream
- 125 ml mayonnaise
- 3 tbsps. fresh coriander (chopped)
- 2 tbsp ranch seasoning
- 2 tbsps. double cream
- 2 tbsps. lime juice
- 1 garlic clove, minced
- salt and pepper

Preparation:

1 Cut veggies to desired size and arrange evenly on a serving platter.
2 Cut turkey into strips and place over the veggies. Scatter the green olives on top.
3 Mix all dressing ingredients until well combined. Drizzle over the salad. Enjoy!

Lunch

One-pot roasted chicken thighs and swede

Dinner

Crock-pot low-carb beef and veggies

Breakfast

Low-carb pancakes

Lunch

Baked celery root with gorgonzola

Time: 50 minutes | Serves: 4

Net carbs: 13 g | Fibre: 4 g | Fat: 36 g | Protein: 12 g | Kcal: 428

Ingredients:

- 3 tbsp olive oil
- 450 g celery root (roots removed, peeled, cut into ½-inch slices)
- salt and pepper
- 75 ml hazelnuts
- 75g baby spinach
- 1red onion (julienned)
- 150 g blue cheese (crumbled)
- 3tbsps. butter
- 75 g mushrooms (quartered)

Preparation:

1   Heat your oven to 200°C (400°F). Line a baking tray with baking sheet.

2   Place the celery root slices onto the baking sheet. Brush the celery slices with the olive oil. Season to taste. Transfer to oven and bake for 40-45 minutes. Remove from oven.

3   Meanwhile, heat butter in a medium-sized frying pan over moderate heat. Add the quartered mushrooms and sauté until soft and golden. Season to taste. Remove from heat.

4   Add the nuts to a dry frying pan and fry them quickly over high heat until fragrant. Remove from pan. Set aside to cool. Chop to desired size.

5   In a salad bowl, toss the spinach leaves, fried mushrooms, sliced onions, and chopped hazelnuts. Mix to combine.

6   Arrange celery root slices on plates. Top with the hazelnut and mushroom salad. Place the blue cheese crumbles over the salad.

Dinner

Low-carb cheesy minced beef wraps

Breakfast

Beef, eggs, and cheese morning casserole

Lunch

Low-carb creamy Tuscan chicken

Dinner

Low-carb ham and cheese pie

Time: 1h25 minutes | Serves: 6
Net carbs: 4 g | Fibre: 1 g | Fat: 20 g | Protein: 21 g | Kcal: 281

Ingredients:

Crust
- ◆350 g cauliflower rice
- ◆1 large egg
- ◆125 ml grated parmesan cheese
- ◆Salt and pepper

Filling
- ◆110 g grated cheddar cheese

- ◆175 g smoked ham
- ◆75 ml double cream
- ◆2 garlic cloves, minced
- ◆5 large free-range eggs
- ◆salt and pepper

Preparation:

1 Heat your oven to 175°C (350°F). Grease a ceramic pie plate.

2 *Pie crust:* Cook the cauliflower rice in a microwave-safe container for 10 minutes until soft. Drain the cauliflower rice by placing it in a tea towel and squeezing it until the liquid has all drained.

3 Place the cauliflower rice into a bowl. Add egg and parmesan and mix to combine. Season to taste. Transfer mixture to the greased ceramic plate and press it into the sides and bottom in a uniform layer. Place in oven. Let cook for 15 min. Remove from oven but maintain oven heat.

4 *Filling:* Whisk all filling ingredients except cheddar and ham until well combined. Place ham on the cauliflower crust. Sprinkle the cheddar cheese over the ham. Add the egg, cream, and garlic mixture. Season to taste. Transfer to oven and bake for 45 minutes longer. It should be set in the centre.

5 Remove from oven. Allow 15-20 minutes to cool before transferring to plates. *Enjoy!*

Breakfast

Brie and nuts low-carb salad

Time: 5 minutes | Serves: 2
Net carbs: 4 g | Fibre: 7 g | Fat: 85 g | Protein: 35 g | Kcal: 936

Ingredients:

- ◆ 110 g salami
- ◆ 200 g Brie cheese
- ◆ 1avocado
- ◆ 40g macadamia nuts
- ◆ 50 g lettuce
- ◆ 30 ml olive oil

Preparation:

1   Mix all ingredients in a bowl. Enjoy!

Lunch

Low-carb ham and cheese sandwich

Dinner

Cauliflower and cheese casserole

Breakfast

Comforting Pumpkin Soup

Lunch

Salmon and prawn salad with mayo dressing

Time: 20 minutes | Serves: 6

Net carbs: 3 g | Fibre: 1 g | Fat: 30 g | Protein: 27 g | Kcal: 394

Ingredients:

- ♦ 450 g cooked prawns (chopped)
- ♦ 450 g cooked salmon (flaked)
- ♦ 1 avocado (pitted, diced)
- ♦ 75 g tomatoes (chopped)
- ♦ 75 g cucumber (diced)

Dressing:
- ♦ 2 tbsps. lime juice
- ♦ 75 ml crème fraiche
- ♦ 125 ml mayonnaise
- ♦ 1 garlic clove (minced)
- ♦ Salt and pepper
- ♦ 60 g red onions (minced)

Preparation:

1. Dressing: Mix all dressing ingredients until well combined. Set aside.
2. Place the prawns, salmon, avocado, tomatoes, and cucumber in a bowl. Toss to combine.
3. Add the dressing over the salad ingredients. Mix to combine. Place in the fridge for 20 to 30 minutes and then serve!

Dinner

Crock-pot low-carb beef and veggies

Breakfast

   Hearty avocado salad

Lunch

   Low-carb beef goulash

Dinner

   Oven-cooked garam masala chicken

Time: 25 minutes | Serves: 4

Net carbs: 6 g | Fibre: 4 g | Fat: 51 g | Protein: 38 g | Kcal: 629

Ingredients:

- ♦ 3 tbsps. butter
- ♦ 650 g chicken breasts
- ♦ Salt
- ♦ 2 ½ tbsps. garam masala (divided)
- ♦ 300 ml double cream
- ♦ 1 red bell pepper (diced)
- ♦ Freshly chopped parsley

Preparation:

1   Heat your oven to 200°C (400°F). Use a sharp knife to cut the chicken breasts in half lengthwise. Season the pieces with salt on both sides.

2   Heat butter in a medium-sized oven-proof frying pan over moderate heat. Place chicken onto the pan and sear on both sides until golden. Stir in ½ of the garam masala. Stir to combine.

3   In a small bowl, mix bell pepper and double cream with remaining garam masala. Pour over the chicken as evenly as possible. Transfer pan to oven and let cook for 20 minutes. Remove from oven.

4   Serve hot with freshly chopped parsley.

Picture: Yaruniv Studios

Julia Sophie Harris by proxy of:

Rocka Maldini

Roka Maldini

120, Old Railway Track

SVR 9017

Santa Venera

Malta

Malta

malta.publishing@gmail.com

IMPRINT

Made in the USA
Lexington, KY
18 August 2019